This journal belongs to:

_____

_____

Self-reflection and Introspection

She stands in front of the mirror's gaze,
A hushed storm with a glowing blaze.
Her scars, body, and stretch marks on her skin
All signs of her battles fought within.
Each perceived flaw is a story, each facial line a song,
An outline of where she's traveled long.
She has learned to see beyond her veil,
Every perceived "flaw" has its own story to tell.
Her crown is heavy, which causes her head to ache,
Nevertheless, her spirit does not break.
She has learned to relax, breathe, and mend,
for self-care is her best friend.
In the stolen hours, she finds her peace,
A sacred pause, a sweet release.
Through the fragrance of candle's glow and the shower's soothing streams.
She heals herself and fuels her dreams.
No need for society's perfection's cruel disguise,
Her beauty lives in her own eyes.
She loves herself, both strong and weak,
A woman whole, both gentle and meek.
So, here's to her—flaws, strength, and grace,
A masterpiece no one can replace.
For in her heart, she holds the key:
To love herself is to be free.

~ Geletta Shavers, LCWS

30 DAY Self-Care Challenge

DAY 1	DAY 2	DAY 3	DAY 4	DAY 5
Pray or Mediate	Eat healthy meals	Spend the day social media free	Call someone you love	Take a 30 minute walk
DAY 6	**DAY 7**	**DAY 8**	**DAY 9**	**DAY 10**
Take a bubble bath or hot shower	Wear your favorite outfit	Stretch for 10-15 minutes	Watch your favorite TV show	Unplug from phone, email, and texts
DAY 11	**DAY 12**	**DAY 13**	**DAY 14**	**DAY 15**
Spend time with positive people	Read a book for 20 minutes	Write a list of short-term goals	De-clutter your environment	Dance, swim, walk, or run
DAY 16	**DAY 17**	**DAY 18**	**DAY 19**	**DAY 20**
Have a game night	Practice self-reflection	Make your favorite meal	Turn off upsetting news	Take yourself out for a date
DAY 21	**DAY 22**	**DAY 23**	**DAY 24**	**DAY 25**
Watch a movie or series	Read a book on self-care	Make a gratitude list	Face one thing you have been avoiding	Take a day trip or staycation
DAY 26	**DAY 27**	**DAY 28**	**DAY 29**	**DAY 30**
Call your family	Spend some time outside	Say 'no' when necessary	Do something safe and fun	Try a new activity

"Self-care is loving yourself and intentionally devoting time to your well-being by being kind to yourself, establishing boundaries, and learning it's okay to say "no!"

When practicing self-care, you are paying attention to YOU!

Self-care techniques
Self-reflection and Introspection
Practice gratitude
Stay positive
Surround yourself with positive people
Eat nutritious meals and snacks
Make yourself a priority
Practice mindfulness skills
Strength and aerobic exercises
Set realistic and achievable goals
Connect with your Higher Power
Adequate sleep
Good hygiene
Yoga/stretching

A daily positive mantra

I will only fill my mind with positive and nourishing thoughts.

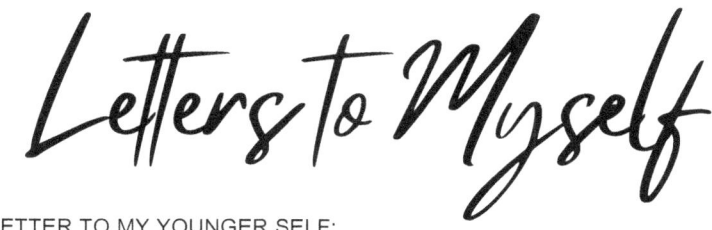

A LETTER TO MY YOUNGER SELF:

_____
_____
_____
_____
_____
_____

A LETTER TO MY CURRENT SELF:

_____
_____
_____
_____
_____
_____

A LETTER TO MY FUTURE SELF:

_____
_____
_____
_____
_____
_____

DAILY SELF-CARE

Date _____ / _____ / _____

MO TU WE TH FR SA SU

My sleep last night was

Approx. hours _____

Get up time _____

Cups of water 💧 💧 💧 💧 💧

Eye exercises 👁 👁 👁

Day to do list

- Brush teeth and wash face
- Eat breakfast and lunch
- Move my body or take a walk
- Get done work tasks
- Open a window and get fresh air
- Time off screens

Evening to do list

- Read 20 pages of a book
- Write to my journal
- Meditate for 10 minutes
- Workout for 30 minutes
- Brush teeth and wash face
- Take a shower

How I was feeling today

_____
_____
_____

SELF-CARE JOURNALING

Today I felt

_____
_____
_____

Today I needed

_____
_____
_____

Date:

DAILY SELF-CARE

Date ___ / ___ / ___

MO TU WE TH FR SA SU

My sleep last night was

♥♥ ☺ 😐 ☹ 😢

Approx. hours _____   Get up time _____

Cups of water 💧 💧 💧 💧 💧

Eye exercises 👁 👁 👁

Day to do list

- Brush teeth and wash face
- Eat breakfast and lunch
- Move my body or take a walk
- Get done work tasks
- Open a window and get fresh air
- Time off screens

Evening to do list

- Read 20 pages of a book
- Write to my journal
- Meditate for 10 minutes
- Workout for 30 minutes
- Brush teeth and wash face
- Take a shower

How I was feeling today

♥♥ ☺ 😐 ☹ 😢

_____
_____
_____
_____

SELF-CARE JOURNALING

Today I felt

_____
_____
_____

Today I needed

_____
_____
_____

Date:

_____
_____
_____
_____
_____
_____
_____
_____
_____
_____
_____
_____
_____
_____

DAILY SELF-CARE

Date _____ / _____ / _____

MO TU WE TH FR SA SU

My sleep last night was   Approx. hours _____   Get up time _____

♥‿♥ ☺ 😐 ☹ 😢

Cups of water 💧 💧 💧 💧 💧   Eye exercises 👁 👁 👁

Day to do list

- Brush teeth and wash face
- Eat breakfast and lunch
- Move my body or take a walk
- Get done work tasks
- Open a window and get fresh air
- Time off screens

Evening to do list

- Read 20 pages of a book
- Write to my journal
- Meditate for 10 minutes
- Workout for 30 minutes
- Brush teeth and wash face
- Take a shower

How I was feeling today

♥‿♥ ☺ 😐 ☹ 😢

_____
_____
_____

SELF-CARE JOURNALING

Today I felt

Today I needed

Date:

DAILY SELF-CARE

Date ____ / ____ / ____

MO TU WE TH FR SA SU

My sleep last night was

Approx. hours _____   Get up time _____

Cups of water ○ ○ ○ ○ ○   Eye exercises ◉ ◉ ◉

Day to do list

- Brush teeth and wash face
- Eat breakfast and lunch
- Move my body or take a walk
- Get done work tasks
- Open a window and get fresh air
- Time off screens

Evening to do list

- Read 20 pages of a book
- Write to my journal
- Meditate for 10 minutes
- Workout for 30 minutes
- Brush teeth and wash face
- Take a shower

How I was feeling today

_____
_____
_____

SELF-CARE JOURNALING

Today I felt

_____
_____
_____

Today I needed

_____
_____
_____

Date:

_____
_____
_____
_____
_____
_____
_____
_____
_____
_____
_____
_____
_____
_____

DAILY SELF-CARE

Date ___ / ___ / ___

MO TU WE TH FR SA SU

My sleep last night was

♥ ☺ 😐 😕 😢

Approx. hours _____

Get up time _____

Cups of water 💧 💧 💧 💧 💧

Eye exercises 👁 👁 👁

Day to do list

- Brush teeth and wash face
- Eat breakfast and lunch
- Move my body or take a walk
- Get done work tasks
- Open a window and get fresh air
- Time off screens

Evening to do list

- Read 20 pages of a book
- Write to my journal
- Meditate for 10 minutes
- Workout for 30 minutes
- Brush teeth and wash face
- Take a shower

How I was feeling today

♥ ☺ 😐 😕 😢

_____
_____
_____

SELF-CARE JOURNALING

Today I felt

_____
_____
_____

Today I needed

_____
_____
_____

Date:

_____
_____
_____
_____
_____
_____
_____
_____
_____
_____
_____
_____
_____
_____

DAILY SELF-CARE

Date ____/____/____

MO TU WE TH FR SA SU

My sleep last night was

😍 🙂 😐 🙁 😢

Approx. hours _____

Get up time _____

Cups of water 💧 💧 💧 💧 💧

Eye exercises 👁 👁 👁

Day to do list

- Brush teeth and wash face
- Eat breakfast and lunch
- Move my body or take a walk
- Get done work tasks
- Open a window and get fresh air
- Time off screens

Evening to do list

- Read 20 pages of a book
- Write to my journal
- Meditate for 10 minutes
- Workout for 30 minutes
- Brush teeth and wash face
- Take a shower

How I was feeling today

😍 🙂 😐 🙁 😢

_____
_____
_____
_____

SELF-CARE JOURNALING

Today I felt

_____
_____
_____

Today I needed

_____
_____
_____

Date:

_____
_____
_____
_____
_____
_____
_____
_____
_____
_____
_____
_____
_____
_____

DAILY SELF-CARE

Date ____/____/____

MO TU WE TH FR SA SU

My sleep last night was   Approx. hours _____   Get up time _____

♥‿♥   ☺   :| :(:,(

Cups of water 💧 💧 💧 💧 💧   Eye exercises 👁 👁 👁

Day to do list

- Brush teeth and wash face
- Eat breakfast and lunch
- Move my body or take a walk
- Get done work tasks
- Open a window and get fresh air
- Time off screens

Evening to do list

- Read 20 pages of a book
- Write to my journal
- Meditate for 10 minutes
- Workout for 30 minutes
- Brush teeth and wash face
- Take a shower

How I was feeling today

♥‿♥   ☺   :| :(:,(

_____
_____
_____

SELF-CARE JOURNALING

Today I felt

_____
_____
_____

Today I needed

_____
_____
_____

Date:

DAILY SELF-CARE

Date _____ / _____ / _____

MO TU WE TH FR SA SU

My sleep last night was

♥♥ ☺ ☹ ☹ ☹

Approx. hours _____   Get up time _____

Cups of water ♦ ♦ ♦ ♦ ♦   Eye exercises ◉ ◉ ◉

Day to do list

- Brush teeth and wash face
- Eat breakfast and lunch
- Move my body or take a walk
- Get done work tasks
- Open a window and get fresh air
- Time off screens

Evening to do list

- Read 20 pages of a book
- Write to my journal
- Meditate for 10 minutes
- Workout for 30 minutes
- Brush teeth and wash face
- Take a shower

How I was feeling today

♥♥ ☺ ☹ ☹ ☹

_____
_____
_____

SELF-CARE JOURNALING

Today I felt

_____
_____
_____

Today I needed

_____
_____
_____

Date:

_____
_____
_____
_____
_____
_____
_____
_____
_____
_____
_____
_____
_____
_____

DAILY SELF-CARE

Date ___/___/___

MO TU WE TH FR SA SU

My sleep last night was

♥♥ ☺ 😐 ☹ 😢

Approx. hours _____

Get up time _____

Cups of water 💧 💧 💧 💧 💧

Eye exercises 👁 👁 👁

Day to do list

- Brush teeth and wash face
- Eat breakfast and lunch
- Move my body or take a walk
- Get done work tasks
- Open a window and get fresh air
- Time off screens

Evening to do list

- Read 20 pages of a book
- Write to my journal
- Meditate for 10 minutes
- Workout for 30 minutes
- Brush teeth and wash face
- Take a shower

How I was feeling today

♥♥ ☺ 😐 ☹ 😢

_____
_____
_____
_____

SELF-CARE JOURNALING

Today I felt

_____
_____
_____

Today I needed

_____
_____
_____

Date:

DAILY SELF-CARE

Date _____ / _____ / _____

MO TU WE TH FR SA SU

My sleep last night was

Approx. hours _____

Get up time _____

Cups of water 💧 💧 💧 💧 💧

Eye exercises 👁 👁 👁

Day to do list

- Brush teeth and wash face
- Eat breakfast and lunch
- Move my body or take a walk
- Get done work tasks
- Open a window and get fresh air
- Time off screens

Evening to do list

- Read 20 pages of a book
- Write to my journal
- Meditate for 10 minutes
- Workout for 30 minutes
- Brush teeth and wash face
- Take a shower

How I was feeling today

_____
_____
_____

SELF-CARE JOURNALING

Today I felt
_____
_____
_____

Today I needed
_____
_____
_____

Date:

_____
_____
_____
_____
_____
_____
_____
_____
_____
_____
_____
_____
_____
_____

DAILY SELF-CARE

Date ___ / ___ / ___

MO TU WE TH FR SA SU

My sleep last night was

♥♥ ☺ 😐 😕 😞

Approx. hours _____

Get up time _____

Cups of water 💧 💧 💧 💧 💧

Eye exercises 👁 👁 👁

Day to do list

- Brush teeth and wash face
- Eat breakfast and lunch
- Move my body or take a walk
- Get done work tasks
- Open a window and get fresh air
- Time off screens

Evening to do list

- Read 20 pages of a book
- Write to my journal
- Meditate for 10 minutes
- Workout for 30 minutes
- Brush teeth and wash face
- Take a shower

How I was feeling today

♥♥ ☺ 😐 😕 😞

_____
_____
_____
_____

SELF-CARE JOURNALING

Today I felt

_____
_____
_____

Today I needed

_____
_____
_____

Date:

DAILY SELF-CARE

Date ___ / ___ / ___

MO TU WE TH FR SA SU

My sleep last night was   Approx. hours _____   Get up time _____

Cups of water   ● ● ● ● ●   Eye exercises 👁 👁 👁

Day to do list

- Brush teeth and wash face
- Eat breakfast and lunch
- Move my body or take a walk
- Get done work tasks
- Open a window and get fresh air
- Time off screens

Evening to do list

- Read 20 pages of a book
- Write to my journal
- Meditate for 10 minutes
- Workout for 30 minutes
- Brush teeth and wash face
- Take a shower

How I was feeling today

_____
_____
_____

SELF-CARE JOURNALING

Today I felt

_____
_____
_____

Today I needed

_____
_____
_____

Date:

_____
_____
_____
_____
_____
_____
_____
_____
_____
_____
_____
_____
_____

DAILY SELF-CARE

Date ___/___/___
MO TU WE TH FR SA SU

My sleep last night was   Approx. hours _____   Get up time _____

♥ ☺ 😐 ☹ 😢

Cups of water 💧 💧 💧 💧 💧   Eye exercises 👁 👁 👁

Day to do list

- Brush teeth and wash face
- Eat breakfast and lunch
- Move my body or take a walk
- Get done work tasks
- Open a window and get fresh air
- Time off screens

Evening to do list

- Read 20 pages of a book
- Write to my journal
- Meditate for 10 minutes
- Workout for 30 minutes
- Brush teeth and wash face
- Take a shower

How I was feeling today

♥ ☺ 😐 ☹ 😢

_____
_____
_____

SELF-CARE JOURNALING

Today I felt

_____
_____
_____

Today I needed

_____
_____
_____

Date:

DAILY SELF-CARE

Date ___ / ___ / ___

MO TU WE TH FR SA SU

My sleep last night was

♥♥ ☺ 😐 ☹ 😢

Approx. hours _____   Get up time _____

Cups of water 💧 💧 💧 💧 💧

Eye exercises 👁 👁 👁

Day to do list

- Brush teeth and wash face
- Eat breakfast and lunch
- Move my body or take a walk
- Get done work tasks
- Open a window and get fresh air
- Time off screens

Evening to do list

- Read 20 pages of a book
- Write to my journal
- Meditate for 10 minutes
- Workout for 30 minutes
- Brush teeth and wash face
- Take a shower

How I was feeling today

♥♥ ☺ 😐 ☹ 😢

_____
_____
_____

SELF-CARE JOURNALING

Today I felt

_____
_____
_____

Today I needed

_____
_____
_____

Date:

DAILY SELF-CARE

Date ___/___/___

MO TU WE TH FR SA SU

My sleep last night was

♥♥ ☺ ☹ ✖ ✖•

Approx. hours _____

Get up time _____

Cups of water ○ ○ ○ ○ ○

Eye exercises ◉ ◉ ◉

Day to do list

- Brush teeth and wash face
- Eat breakfast and lunch
- Move my body or take a walk
- Get done work tasks
- Open a window and get fresh air
- Time off screens

Evening to do list

- Read 20 pages of a book
- Write to my journal
- Meditate for 10 minutes
- Workout for 30 minutes
- Brush teeth and wash face
- Take a shower

How I was feeling today

♥♥ ☺ ☹ ✖ ✖•

_____
_____
_____
_____

SELF-CARE JOURNALING

Today I felt

_____
_____
_____

Today I needed

_____
_____
_____

Date:

_____
_____
_____
_____
_____
_____
_____
_____
_____
_____
_____
_____
_____
_____

DAILY SELF-CARE

Date ___ / ___ / ___

MO TU WE TH FR SA SU

My sleep last night was

Approx. hours _____ Get up time _____

Cups of water 💧 💧 💧 💧 💧

Eye exercises 👁 👁 👁

Day to do list

- Brush teeth and wash face
- Eat breakfast and lunch
- Move my body or take a walk
- Get done work tasks
- Open a window and get fresh air
- Time off screens

Evening to do list

- Read 20 pages of a book
- Write to my journal
- Meditate for 10 minutes
- Workout for 30 minutes
- Brush teeth and wash face
- Take a shower

How I was feeling today

_____
_____
_____
_____

SELF-CARE JOURNALING

Today I felt

_____
_____
_____

Today I needed

_____
_____
_____

Date:

DAILY SELF-CARE

Date ___/___/___

MO TU WE TH FR SA SU

My sleep last night was

♥♥ ☺ ☹ ☹ ☹

Approx. hours _____

Get up time _____

Cups of water 💧 💧 💧 💧 💧

Eye exercises 👁 👁 👁

Day to do list

- Brush teeth and wash face
- Eat breakfast and lunch
- Move my body or take a walk
- Get done work tasks
- Open a window and get fresh air
- Time off screens

Evening to do list

- Read 20 pages of a book
- Write to my journal
- Meditate for 10 minutes
- Workout for 30 minutes
- Brush teeth and wash face
- Take a shower

How I was feeling today

♥♥ ☺ ☹ ☹ ☹

_____

_____

_____

SELF-CARE JOURNALING

(Today I felt)

_____
_____
_____

(Today I needed)

_____
_____
_____

Date:

_____
_____
_____
_____
_____
_____
_____
_____
_____
_____
_____
_____
_____
_____

DAILY SELF-CARE

Date ___ / ___ / ___

MO TU WE TH FR SA SU

My sleep last night was

Approx. hours _____   Get up time _____

Cups of water 💧 💧 💧 💧 💧   Eye exercises 👁 👁 👁

Day to do list

- Brush teeth and wash face
- Eat breakfast and lunch
- Move my body or take a walk
- Get done work tasks
- Open a window and get fresh air
- Time off screens

Evening to do list

- Read 20 pages of a book
- Write to my journal
- Meditate for 10 minutes
- Workout for 30 minutes
- Brush teeth and wash face
- Take a shower

How I was feeling today

_____
_____
_____

SELF-CARE JOURNALING

Today I felt

_____
_____
_____

Today I needed

_____
_____
_____

Date:

DAILY SELF-CARE

Date _____ / _____ / _____

MO TU WE TH FR SA SU

My sleep last night was

Approx. hours _____

Get up time _____

Cups of water 💧 💧 💧 💧 💧

Eye exercises 👁 👁 👁

Day to do list

- Brush teeth and wash face
- Eat breakfast and lunch
- Move my body or take a walk
- Get done work tasks
- Open a window and get fresh air
- Time off screens

Evening to do list

- Read 20 pages of a book
- Write to my journal
- Meditate for 10 minutes
- Workout for 30 minutes
- Brush teeth and wash face
- Take a shower

How I was feeling today

_____
_____
_____

SELF-CARE JOURNALING

Today I felt

_____
_____
_____

Today I needed

_____
_____
_____

Date:

DAILY SELF-CARE

Date ____/____/____

MO TU WE TH FR SA SU

My sleep last night was

Approx. hours _____   Get up time _____

Cups of water 💧 💧 💧 💧 💧   Eye exercises 👁 👁 👁

Day to do list

- Brush teeth and wash face
- Eat breakfast and lunch
- Move my body or take a walk
- Get done work tasks
- Open a window and get fresh air
- Time off screens

Evening to do list

- Read 20 pages of a book
- Write to my journal
- Meditate for 10 minutes
- Workout for 30 minutes
- Brush teeth and wash face
- Take a shower

How I was feeling today

_____
_____
_____

SELF-CARE JOURNALING

Today I felt

_____
_____
_____

Today I needed

_____
_____
_____

Date:

_____
_____
_____
_____
_____
_____
_____
_____
_____
_____
_____
_____
_____
_____
_____

DAILY SELF-CARE

Date ____/____/____

MO TU WE TH FR SA SU

My sleep last night was

Approx. hours _____   Get up time _____

Cups of water   ● ● ● ● ●   Eye exercises   ◉ ◉ ◉

Day to do list

- Brush teeth and wash face
- Eat breakfast and lunch
- Move my body or take a walk
- Get done work tasks
- Open a window and get fresh air
- Time off screens

Evening to do list

- Read 20 pages of a book
- Write to my journal
- Meditate for 10 minutes
- Workout for 30 minutes
- Brush teeth and wash face
- Take a shower

How I was feeling today

_____
_____
_____

SELF-CARE JOURNALING

Today I felt

_____
_____
_____

Today I needed

_____
_____
_____

Date:

_____
_____
_____
_____
_____
_____
_____
_____
_____
_____
_____
_____
_____
_____

DAILY SELF-CARE

Date ____ / ____ / ____

MO TU WE TH FR SA SU

My sleep last night was

Approx. hours _____   Get up time _____

Cups of water 💧 💧 💧 💧 💧   Eye exercises 👁 👁 👁

Day to do list

- Brush teeth and wash face
- Eat breakfast and lunch
- Move my body or take a walk
- Get done work tasks
- Open a window and get fresh air
- Time off screens

Evening to do list

- Read 20 pages of a book
- Write to my journal
- Meditate for 10 minutes
- Workout for 30 minutes
- Brush teeth and wash face
- Take a shower

How I was feeling today

_____
_____
_____

SELF-CARE JOURNALING

Today I felt

_____
_____
_____

Today I needed

_____
_____
_____

Date:

DAILY SELF-CARE

Date ___ / ___ / ___

MO TU WE TH FR SA SU

My sleep last night was   Approx. hours _____   Get up time _____

Cups of water 💧 💧 💧 💧 💧   Eye exercises 👁 👁 👁

Day to do list

- Brush teeth and wash face
- Eat breakfast and lunch
- Move my body or take a walk
- Get done work tasks
- Open a window and get fresh air
- Time off screens

Evening to do list

- Read 20 pages of a book
- Write to my journal
- Meditate for 10 minutes
- Workout for 30 minutes
- Brush teeth and wash face
- Take a shower

How I was feeling today

SELF-CARE JOURNALING

Today I felt

_____
_____
_____

Today I needed

_____
_____
_____

Date:

DAILY SELF-CARE

Date ____ / ____ / ____

MO TU WE TH FR SA SU

My sleep last night was

😍 🙂 😐 😕 😢

Approx. hours _____

Get up time _____

Cups of water 💧 💧 💧 💧 💧

Eye exercises 👁 👁 👁

Day to do list

- Brush teeth and wash face
- Eat breakfast and lunch
- Move my body or take a walk
- Get done work tasks
- Open a window and get fresh air
- Time off screens

Evening to do list

- Read 20 pages of a book
- Write to my journal
- Meditate for 10 minutes
- Workout for 30 minutes
- Brush teeth and wash face
- Take a shower

How I was feeling today

😍 🙂 😐 😕 😢

_____
_____
_____

SELF-CARE JOURNALING

Today I felt

_____
_____
_____

Today I needed

_____
_____
_____

Date:

DAILY SELF-CARE

Date ___/___/___

MO TU WE TH FR SA SU

My sleep last night was

♥♥ ☺ ☹ ☹ ☹

Approx. hours _____

Get up time _____

Cups of water 💧 💧 💧 💧 💧

Eye exercises 👁 👁 👁

Day to do list

- Brush teeth and wash face
- Eat breakfast and lunch
- Move my body or take a walk
- Get done work tasks
- Open a window and get fresh air
- Time off screens

Evening to do list

- Read 20 pages of a book
- Write to my journal
- Meditate for 10 minutes
- Workout for 30 minutes
- Brush teeth and wash face
- Take a shower

How I was feeling today

♥♥ ☺ ☹ ☹ ☹

_____
_____
_____

SELF-CARE JOURNALING

Today I felt

_____
_____
_____

Today I needed

_____
_____
_____

Date:

DAILY SELF-CARE

Date ___/___/___

MO TU WE TH FR SA SU

My sleep last night was   Approx. hours _____   Get up time _____

♥♥ ☺ ☹ ☹ 😢

Cups of water 💧 💧 💧 💧 💧   Eye exercises 👁 👁 👁

Day to do list

- Brush teeth and wash face
- Eat breakfast and lunch
- Move my body or take a walk
- Get done work tasks
- Open a window and get fresh air
- Time off screens

Evening to do list

- Read 20 pages of a book
- Write to my journal
- Meditate for 10 minutes
- Workout for 30 minutes
- Brush teeth and wash face
- Take a shower

How I was feeling today

♥♥ ☺ ☹ ☹ 😢

_____
_____
_____

SELF-CARE JOURNALING

Today I felt

_____
_____
_____

Today I needed

_____
_____
_____

Date:

DAILY SELF-CARE

Date ___ / ___ / ___

MO TU WE TH FR SA SU

My sleep last night was

Approx. hours _____   Get up time _____

Cups of water 💧 💧 💧 💧 💧   Eye exercises 👁 👁 👁

Day to do list

- Brush teeth and wash face
- Eat breakfast and lunch
- Move my body or take a walk
- Get done work tasks
- Open a window and get fresh air
- Time off screens

Evening to do list

- Read 20 pages of a book
- Write to my journal
- Meditate for 10 minutes
- Workout for 30 minutes
- Brush teeth and wash face
- Take a shower

How I was feeling today

_____
_____
_____

SELF-CARE JOURNALING

Today I felt

_____
_____
_____

Today I needed

_____
_____
_____

Date:

DAILY SELF-CARE

Date ___ / ___ / ___

MO TU WE TH FR SA SU

My sleep last night was

Approx. hours _____   Get up time _____

Cups of water 💧 💧 💧 💧 💧

Eye exercises 👁 👁 👁

Day to do list

- Brush teeth and wash face
- Eat breakfast and lunch
- Move my body or take a walk
- Get done work tasks
- Open a window and get fresh air
- Time off screens

Evening to do list

- Read 20 pages of a book
- Write to my journal
- Meditate for 10 minutes
- Workout for 30 minutes
- Brush teeth and wash face
- Take a shower

How I was feeling today

_____
_____
_____

SELF-CARE JOURNALING

Today I felt

_____
_____
_____

Today I needed

_____
_____
_____

Date:

_____
_____
_____
_____
_____
_____
_____
_____
_____
_____
_____
_____
_____
_____
_____

DAILY SELF-CARE

Date _____ / _____ / _____

MO TU WE TH FR SA SU

My sleep last night was

Approx. hours _____   Get up time _____

Cups of water 💧 💧 💧 💧 💧   Eye exercises 👁 👁 👁

Day to do list

- Brush teeth and wash face
- Eat breakfast and lunch
- Move my body or take a walk
- Get done work tasks
- Open a window and get fresh air
- Time off screens

Evening to do list

- Read 20 pages of a book
- Write to my journal
- Meditate for 10 minutes
- Workout for 30 minutes
- Brush teeth and wash face
- Take a shower

How I was feeling today

_____
_____
_____

SELF-CARE JOURNALING

Today I felt	Today I needed
_____	_____
_____	_____
_____	_____

Date:

DAILY SELF-CARE

Date ___ / ___ / ___

MO TU WE TH FR SA SU

My sleep last night was

Approx. hours _____   Get up time _____

Cups of water ● ● ● ● ●   Eye exercises 👁 👁 👁

Day to do list

- Brush teeth and wash face
- Eat breakfast and lunch
- Move my body or take a walk
- Get done work tasks
- Open a window and get fresh air
- Time off screens

Evening to do list

- Read 20 pages of a book
- Write to my journal
- Meditate for 10 minutes
- Workout for 30 minutes
- Brush teeth and wash face
- Take a shower

How I was feeling today

_____
_____
_____
_____

SELF-CARE JOURNALING

(Today I felt) (Today I needed)

_____ _____
_____ _____
_____ _____

Date:

_____
_____
_____
_____
_____
_____
_____
_____
_____
_____
_____
_____
_____
_____
_____
_____

DAILY SELF-CARE

Date ____ / ____ / ____

MO TU WE TH FR SA SU

My sleep last night was

😍 🙂 😐 😕 😢

Approx. hours _____

Get up time _____

Cups of water 💧 💧 💧 💧 💧

Eye exercises 👁 👁 👁

Day to do list

- Brush teeth and wash face
- Eat breakfast and lunch
- Move my body or take a walk
- Get done work tasks
- Open a window and get fresh air
- Time off screens

Evening to do list

- Read 20 pages of a book
- Write to my journal
- Meditate for 10 minutes
- Workout for 30 minutes
- Brush teeth and wash face
- Take a shower

How I was feeling today

😍 🙂 😐 😕 😢

_____
_____
_____

SELF-CARE JOURNALING

Today I felt

_____
_____
_____

Today I needed

_____
_____
_____

Date:

daily journal   **DATE**   /   /

daily journal   **DATE** / /

daily journal   DATE   /   /

daily journal DATE   /   /

daily journal DATE   /   /

daily journal   DATE   /   /

daily journal   DATE   /   /

daily journal DATE / /

daily journal   **DATE**   /   /

daily journal   **DATE**   /   /

daily journal DATE   /   /

daily journal   **DATE**   /   /

daily journal DATE   /   /

daily journal **DATE** / /

daily journal   DATE   /   /

daily journal DATE   /   /

daily journal DATE   /   /

daily journal   DATE   /   /

daily journal   DATE   /   /

daily journal   DATE   /   /

daily journal   DATE   /   /

daily journal   **DATE**   /   /

daily journal   **DATE**   /   /

daily journal DATE / /

daily journal

DATE   /   /

daily journal DATE   /   /

daily journal

DATE / /

daily journal DATE   /   /

daily journal   DATE   /   /

daily journal DATE   /   /

daily journal   **DATE**   /   /

daily journal　　　DATE　　/　　/

daily journal DATE   /   /

daily journal DATE   /   /

daily journal   DATE   /   /

www.ingramcontent.com/pod-product-compliance
Lightning Source LLC
Chambersburg PA
CBHW052033030426
42337CB00027B/4984